T

Introduction………………………………..2

Sleep…………………………………………..6

Hunger……………………………………..24

Recovery………………………………….36

Energy……………………………………..52

Digestion………………………………….66

Stress……………………………………….78

Strategies for improvement…………92

Develop a Plan……………………………100

Conclusion………………………………….105

Introduction

Sleep, hunger, recovery, energy, digestion, and stress are all essential factors that impact health and fitness. Sleep is critical for physical and mental restoration, hormonal balance, and optimal cognitive functioning. Hunger and nutrition are critical for maintaining a healthy weight, building and repairing muscle, and providing energy for daily activities. Recovery is essential for muscle growth, injury prevention, and overall physical and mental health. Energy is vital for physical activity, mental focus, and general well-being. Digestion is essential for nutrient absorption and waste elimination. Stress, both physical and mental, can have a significant impact on all these factors, affecting appetite, digestion, hormone levels, energy, and sleep.

These factors are all interconnected and can impact each other. Poor sleep quality can increase hunger and cravings, affect metabolism and hormone levels, and reduce energy levels. Hunger and nutrient deficiencies can negatively impact sleep, energy levels, and recovery. Lack of recovery can lead to injury, reduce energy levels, and affect sleep quality. Low energy levels can decrease physical activity and affect digestion and sleep quality. Poor digestion can negatively impact nutrient absorption and energy levels, while stress can affect all these factors, leading to negative health outcomes.

Overall, optimizing sleep, hunger, recovery, energy, digestion, and stress is crucial for maintaining good health and fitness. Understanding the interconnectedness of these factors can help individuals create a personalized plan to improve their health and fitness goals.

Sleep and its impact on health and fitness

Sleep is essential for maintaining optimal physical and mental health. It is a critical process that helps the body and mind to repair, regenerate, and rejuvenate. During sleep, the body repairs damaged tissues, consolidates memories, and releases hormones that regulate various bodily functions. Lack of sleep can cause a range of physical and mental health problems, including weight gain, diabetes, heart disease, depression, anxiety, and impaired cognitive function.

Physical health

Sleep is essential for physical health. It allows the body to repair and regenerate tissues, including muscle, bone, and skin. During sleep, the body releases growth hormones that help to build and repair tissues, increase muscle mass, and strengthen bones. Lack of sleep can affect the body's ability to repair and regenerate, leading to decreased physical performance, increased risk of injury, and delayed recovery from exercise or injury.

Sleep also plays a critical role in maintaining a healthy immune system. During sleep, the body produces cytokines, which help to fight off infection, inflammation, and stress. Lack of sleep can decrease the production of cytokines, making it harder for the body to fight off infections and illnesses.

Mental health

Sleep is also essential for mental health. It plays a critical role in regulating mood, emotions, and cognitive function. During sleep, the brain consolidates memories, processes information, and prepares for the next day's activities. Lack of sleep can lead to cognitive impairment, including decreased concentration, memory, and decision-making ability.

Sleep is also crucial for emotional regulation. Sleep deprivation has been linked to increased levels of stress, anxiety, and depression. Lack of sleep can also increase the risk of developing mood disorders and can exacerbate existing mental health conditions.

Overall, sleep is critical for maintaining optimal physical and mental health. It is essential to prioritize getting enough sleep each night to support overall well-being and prevent the negative health outcomes associated with sleep deprivation.

Sleep is a complex process that is divided into several stages. Each stage of sleep serves a specific function and is characterized by distinct patterns of brain activity, muscle tone, and physiological responses. There are two main types of sleep: Non-REM (NREM) sleep and REM (rapid eye movement) sleep. NREM sleep is further divided into three stages, while REM sleep is a distinct stage.

Stage 1 NREM sleep

Stage 1 NREM sleep is the transition phase between wakefulness and sleep. It is a light sleep stage that lasts for a few minutes and is characterized by slow, rolling eye movements and slowing of brain waves. During this stage, people may experience sudden muscle twitches and may feel as if they are drifting in and out of sleep.

Stage 2 NREM sleep

Stage 2 NREM sleep is a deeper stage of sleep that lasts for about 20 minutes. During this stage, eye movements stop, and brain waves slow down further. Sleep spindles, which are rapid bursts of brain activity, and K-complexes, which are high-amplitude brain waves, occur during this stage. This stage of sleep is essential for consolidating memories and is the longest stage of the sleep cycle.

Stage 3 NREM sleep

Stage 3 NREM sleep, also known as slow-wave sleep or deep sleep, is the stage of sleep that is critical for physical restoration and recovery. It is characterized by slow, delta brain waves and is the deepest stage of sleep. During this stage, the body repairs and regenerates tissues, including muscle and bone, and releases growth hormones. This stage of sleep is also essential for immune function and overall physical health.

REM sleep

REM sleep is the stage of sleep where most dreaming occurs. It is characterized by rapid eye movements, increased brain activity, and muscle paralysis. REM sleep is critical for cognitive function, emotional regulation, and memory consolidation. During REM sleep, the brain processes and consolidates emotional memories and experiences, which is why it is essential for emotional well-being.

The sleep cycle

The sleep cycle is the pattern of alternating NREM and REM sleep stages that occur throughout the night. A typical sleep cycle lasts around 90 minutes, and a complete sleep cycle consists of all stages of sleep. As the night progresses, the duration of REM sleep increases, while the duration of NREM sleep decreases. It is essential to complete a full sleep cycle to feel rested and refreshed in the morning.

Overall, each stage of sleep serves a specific function and is critical for physical and mental health. It is essential to prioritize getting enough sleep each night to support overall well-being and prevent the negative health outcomes associated with sleep deprivation.

Lack of sleep can have a significant impact on appetite, hormone levels, metabolism, and energy levels, leading to negative consequences for overall health and well-being.

Appetite

Sleep deprivation can disrupt the regulation of appetite hormones, leading to increased hunger and food cravings. The hormone leptin, which signals the brain to stop eating when full, decreases with sleep deprivation, while the hormone ghrelin, which signals the brain to eat, increases. This hormonal imbalance can lead to overeating, weight gain, and an increased risk of obesity.

Hormone levels

Sleep plays a crucial role in regulating hormone levels, including those that impact metabolism and energy balance. Lack of sleep can disrupt the natural release of these hormones, leading to imbalances that affect the body's ability to regulate blood sugar levels, burn calories, and manage appetite.

Metabolism

Sleep deprivation can also disrupt metabolism, leading to decreased insulin sensitivity, impaired glucose tolerance, and an increased risk of type 2 diabetes. Additionally, sleep deprivation can decrease the body's ability to metabolize carbohydrates, leading to a shift towards storing energy as fat rather than using it for fuel.

Energy levels

Sleep is essential for restoring energy levels and allowing the body to function optimally. Lack of sleep can lead to decreased alertness, decreased cognitive function, and decreased physical performance. Additionally, chronic sleep deprivation can lead to long-term fatigue, increased risk of accidents and injuries, and decreased quality of life.

Overall, lack of sleep can have a significant impact on appetite, hormone levels, metabolism, and energy levels. It is essential to prioritize getting enough quality sleep each night to support overall health and well-being.

Improving sleep quality can be achieved through several lifestyle changes and habits that promote relaxation, comfort, and a consistent sleep routine. Here are some tips for improving sleep quality:

Establish a regular sleep routine

Go to bed and wake up at the same time each day, even on weekends.

This helps regulate the body's internal clock and promote a consistent sleep-wake cycle.

Create a comfortable sleep environment

Keep your bedroom cool, dark, and quiet. Invest in a comfortable mattress, pillows, and bedding that support your body and keep you comfortable throughout the night.

Limit caffeine and alcohol intake

Caffeine can interfere with falling asleep and staying asleep, so it is best to avoid caffeine-containing foods and drinks, such as coffee, tea, soda, and chocolate, in the evening. Alcohol can also disrupt sleep, so it is best to limit alcohol intake, especially close to bedtime.

Limit screen time before bed

The blue light emitted from electronic devices such as smartphones, tablets, and computers can interfere with sleep by suppressing melatonin, a hormone that regulates sleep-wake cycles. Avoid using electronic devices at least an hour before bedtime.

Relax before bed

Establish a bedtime routine that includes activities that help you relax, such as taking a warm bath, reading a book, practicing relaxation techniques like yoga or meditation, or listening to calming music.

Exercise regularly

Exercise can promote better sleep by reducing stress and anxiety, regulating body temperature, and promoting relaxation. However, it is best to avoid exercising close to bedtime, as it can stimulate the body and make it harder to fall asleep.

Manage stress

Stress and anxiety can interfere with sleep. Consider stress management techniques such as deep breathing, progressive muscle relaxation, or talking to a therapist to manage stress and improve sleep.

By incorporating these tips into your daily routine, you can improve the quality of your sleep and support overall health and well-being.

Hunger and its impact on health and fitness

Hunger and appetite are regulated by a complex interplay of hormones, including ghrelin and leptin.

Ghrelin is a hormone produced by the stomach that stimulates hunger. It is released when the stomach is empty, and its levels rise before meals and fall after eating. Ghrelin signals the brain to increase appetite and to search for food, ultimately leading to food intake. In addition, ghrelin may also influence the body's energy balance, as it can stimulate the release of growth hormone and affect fat storage.

Leptin, on the other hand, is a hormone produced by fat cells that helps regulate appetite and energy balance. Leptin signals the brain to reduce appetite and increase energy expenditure. When fat stores are high, leptin levels increase, signaling the brain to reduce hunger and increase metabolism, ultimately leading to weight loss. In contrast, when fat stores are low, leptin levels decrease, signaling the brain to increase hunger and decrease metabolism, ultimately leading to weight gain.

Both ghrelin and leptin are part of a complex feedback system that helps regulate appetite and energy balance. Ghrelin stimulates hunger and food intake, while leptin helps to suppress appetite and increase energy expenditure. In a healthy individual, these hormones work together to maintain a balance between energy intake and expenditure. However, imbalances in these hormones can lead to disrupted appetite regulation and weight gain or loss.

Factors such as sleep deprivation, stress, and certain medications can disrupt the balance of these hormones, leading to increased hunger and disrupted appetite regulation. Additionally, conditions such as obesity and eating disorders can also impact the regulation of these hormones and lead to abnormal appetite and energy regulation.

Overall, hormones such as ghrelin and leptin play a crucial role in regulating hunger and appetite. Understanding how these hormones work can help individuals make informed choices about their diet and lifestyle to promote healthy appetite regulation and maintain a healthy weight.

The impact of nutrient-dense foods, hydration, and stress management on hunger cues can be significant. By choosing nutrient-dense foods, staying hydrated, and managing stress levels, individuals can help regulate their appetite and reduce the likelihood of overeating or experiencing cravings.

Nutrient-dense foods are those that provide a high amount of nutrients relative to their calorie content.

These include fruits, vegetables, whole grains, lean proteins, and healthy fats. When individuals consume a diet rich in these foods, their bodies receive the nutrients they need to function properly, reducing the likelihood of hunger and cravings. Additionally, these foods are typically lower in calories than processed and junk foods, which can help individuals maintain a healthy weight.

Hydration is also important for regulating hunger cues. Many people mistake thirst for hunger, leading them to consume unnecessary calories when what they really need is water. By staying hydrated, individuals can reduce the likelihood of this confusion and help regulate their appetite. Additionally, drinking water before meals can help individuals feel fuller and reduce the amount of food they consume.

Finally, stress management is important for regulating hunger cues. Stress can trigger the release of hormones such as cortisol, which can increase appetite and lead to overeating. By practicing stress management techniques such as meditation, deep breathing, and exercise, individuals can reduce the impact of stress on their appetite and promote healthy eating habits.

Overall, the impact of nutrient-dense foods, hydration, and stress management on hunger cues can be significant. By choosing a diet rich in nutrient-dense foods, staying hydrated, and managing stress levels, individuals can help regulate their appetite and reduce the likelihood of overeating or experiencing cravings. This can contribute to maintaining a healthy weight and promoting overall health and wellness.

Maintaining a healthy and balanced diet is essential for overall health and well-being. Here are some tips for maintaining a healthy and balanced diet:

Portion control

Eating the right amount of food is key to maintaining a healthy weight. Use smaller plates and avoid going back for seconds. Use your hand to estimate appropriate portions: one serving of protein should be the size of your palm, one serving of carbohydrates should be the size of your fist, and one serving of healthy fats should be the size of your thumb.

Eat a variety of nutrient-dense foods

Focus on incorporating a variety of fruits, vegetables, whole grains, lean proteins, and healthy fats into your diet. These foods provide essential nutrients for your body and can help reduce the risk of chronic diseases.

Mindful eating

Pay attention to your body's hunger cues and eat slowly, savoring each bite. This can help you feel more satisfied and reduce the likelihood of overeating. Avoid distractions such as watching TV or using your phone while eating.

Plan and prepare meals in advance

Plan your meals for the week ahead of time and prepare them in advance. This can help you avoid making unhealthy food choices when you are busy or on-the-go.

Avoid processed and junk foods

These foods are typically high in calories, sugar, and unhealthy fats, and provide little nutritional value. Instead, focus on nutrient-dense whole foods.

Hydrate with water

Drinking enough water is important for maintaining hydration and can also help regulate appetite. Aim for at least 8 glasses of water per day.

Moderation

Enjoy your favorite foods in moderation. All foods can fit into a healthy diet, if they are consumed in moderation and as part of an overall balanced diet.

By incorporating these tips into your daily routine, you can maintain a healthy and balanced diet, promote overall health and well-being, and reduce the risk of chronic diseases.

Recovery and its impact on health and fitness

Recovery is an essential component of physical and mental health. In the context of exercise and fitness, recovery refers to the process by which the body repairs and rebuilds itself after physical activity. This process allows the body to adapt to the stress of exercise and become stronger and more resilient over time. However, recovery is not just important for physical health – it is also essential for mental health and well-being.

Physical Recovery

During physical activity, the body undergoes stress and damage to muscle fibers, which can lead to soreness, fatigue, and decreased performance. Recovery allows the body to repair these damaged tissues, replenish energy stores, and remove waste products such as lactic acid. Proper recovery can also help prevent injuries and overuse injuries that can result from inadequate rest and recovery time.

Mental Recovery

Mental recovery is just as important as physical recovery. Exercise is a stressor on the body, and if not managed properly, it can lead to mental exhaustion, burnout, and decreased motivation. Taking time to rest and recover allows the body and mind to recharge, reducing stress levels and improving overall mental health and well-being. This can lead to increased focus, better mood, and improved cognitive function.

Importance of Sleep for Recovery

Sleep is an essential component of recovery, both for physical and mental health. During sleep, the body repairs and regenerates tissues, releases growth hormones, and restores energy stores. Lack of sleep can disrupt this process, leading to decreased performance, increased risk of injury, and impaired cognitive function. It can also lead to mental health issues such as anxiety and depression.

Importance of Nutrition for Recovery

Nutrition also plays a crucial role in recovery. Adequate intake of protein, carbohydrates, and healthy fats provides the building blocks necessary for tissue repair and regeneration. Proper hydration is also essential for recovery, as it helps to flush out waste products and replenish fluids lost during physical activity.

Overall, recovery is essential for physical and mental health. It allows the body and mind to recharge, repair, and rebuild, leading to improved performance, decreased risk of injury, and improved overall health and well-being. Proper recovery requires adequate sleep, nutrition, and rest time, so it is important to prioritize recovery as part of any fitness or exercise routine.

There are two main types of recovery: active and passive. Both are important for maintaining physical and mental health, but they differ in their approach and benefits.

Active Recovery

Active recovery involves engaging in low-intensity exercise or movement after a period of high-intensity activity. This can help increase blood flow, which in turn promotes the delivery of oxygen and nutrients to the muscles, facilitating the recovery process. Active recovery can also help reduce muscle soreness, stiffness, and inflammation, while improving flexibility and range of motion.

Examples of active recovery include:

- Light jogging or cycling
- Yoga or stretching
- Foam rolling or massage
- Swimming or water aerobics
- Walking or hiking

Passive Recovery

Passive recovery, on the other hand, involves taking a break from physical activity and allowing the body to rest and recover. This can include activities such as sleep, meditation, or simply sitting and relaxing. Passive recovery can be especially important for those engaging in high-intensity or frequent exercise, as it allows the body time to fully recover and rebuild.

Examples of passive recovery include:

- Sleep

- Rest days or taking time off from exercise

- Massage or other bodywork

- Meditation or mindfulness practices

- Spending time in nature or engaging in other stress-reducing activities

Both active and passive recovery have their own unique benefits, and the best approach may vary depending on individual needs and preferences. It is important to listen to your body and prioritize recovery as part of any fitness or exercise routine.

Stress, sleep, and nutrition are all interconnected factors that impact recovery. When one or more of these factors are out of balance, it can negatively affect the body's ability to recover and repair.

Stress

Chronic stress can lead to increased levels of the stress hormone cortisol, which can interfere with the body's ability to recover. High levels of cortisol can lead to muscle breakdown and impaired immune function, which can slow down the recovery process. In order to promote recovery, it is important to manage stress through practices such as meditation, deep breathing, or other stress-reducing activities.

Sleep

Sleep is a crucial component of recovery, as it is during this time that the body repairs and regenerates itself. Lack of sleep or poor sleep quality can lead to increased levels of cortisol and inflammation, both of which can hinder the recovery process. It is important to prioritize sleep and establish a regular sleep routine in order to promote optimal recovery.

<u>Nutrition</u>

Nutrition is another important factor in recovery. Consuming a balanced diet with sufficient protein, carbohydrates, and healthy fats can help support muscle repair and growth. Proper hydration is also crucial for recovery, as dehydration can impair the body's ability to transport nutrients and oxygen to the muscles. It is important to fuel the body with nutrient-dense foods and stay hydrated in order to support the recovery process.

In order to promote optimal recovery, it is important to prioritize and balance all of these interconnected factors. Managing stress, prioritizing sleep, and fueling the body with proper nutrition can all help support the body's ability to recover and repair. Additionally, incorporating active and passive recovery strategies can help further support the recovery process. It is important to listen to your body and prioritize recovery as part of any fitness or exercise routine.

Optimizing recovery is crucial for maximizing the benefits of exercise and physical activity. Here are some tips for optimizing recovery:

Incorporate rest days

Rest days are crucial for allowing the body to recover and repair. It is important to schedule regular rest days and avoid overtraining, which can lead to fatigue, injury, and impaired recovery.

Hydrate properly

Proper hydration is crucial for supporting recovery, as it helps to transport nutrients and oxygen to the muscles. Aim to drink at least 8 cups of water per day and hydrate before, during, and after exercise.

Eat nutrient-dense foods

Consuming a balanced diet with sufficient protein, carbohydrates, and healthy fats can help support muscle repair and growth. Incorporating nutrient-dense foods such as fruits, vegetables, whole grains, and lean protein sources can provide the necessary nutrients to support recovery.

Incorporate active recovery

Active recovery refers to low-intensity exercise or movements that can help to increase blood flow and promote muscle repair. Incorporating activities such as yoga, stretching, or light aerobic exercise can help to promote recovery.

Practice good sleep hygiene

Prioritizing sleep is crucial for recovery, as it is during this time that the body repairs and regenerates itself. Establish a regular sleep routine, avoid caffeine and screen time before bed, and create a comfortable sleep environment to promote optimal sleep.

Manage stress

Chronic stress can interfere with the body's ability to recover. Incorporating stress-reducing activities such as meditation, deep breathing, or other relaxation techniques can help to manage stress and promote recovery.

By prioritizing recovery and incorporating these tips, you can optimize your body's ability to recover and repair, which can ultimately lead to improved physical and mental health.

Energy and its impact on health and fitness

Energy is essential for physical activity and overall health. The human body requires energy to perform basic bodily functions such as breathing, digestion, and circulation, as well as for physical activity and exercise.

Energy is primarily derived from the food we eat, which is broken down and converted into a form of energy known as adenosine triphosphate (ATP). ATP is the primary source of energy used by the body to power muscular contractions during physical activity.

In addition to supporting physical activity, energy is also crucial for overall health. The body requires energy to maintain normal bodily functions, repair and regenerate tissues, and support the immune system.

When the body does not have enough energy, it can result in fatigue, decreased physical performance, and impaired cognitive function. Additionally, chronic low energy levels can lead to a variety of health problems, including nutrient deficiencies, metabolic disorders, and cardiovascular disease.

To maintain optimal energy levels, it is important to consume a balanced diet that provides enough carbohydrates, protein, and healthy fats. Additionally, staying hydrated and getting regular exercise can help to support energy levels and overall health.

In some cases, energy levels may be impacted by underlying medical conditions such as hypothyroidism or anemia. If you are experiencing persistent fatigue or low energy levels, it is important to speak with a healthcare provider to determine the underlying cause and develop an appropriate treatment plan.

Macronutrients, micronutrients, and hydration all play a crucial role in energy production.

Macronutrients are the three major nutrient groups that provide the body with energy: carbohydrates, proteins, and fats. Carbohydrates are the body's primary source of energy and are broken down into glucose, which is used by cells to produce ATP. Proteins can also be broken down into glucose, but their primary role is to repair and maintain tissues in the body. Fats are the most concentrated source of energy and are broken down into fatty acids, which can be used by cells to produce ATP.

Micronutrients, on the other hand, do not provide energy directly, but they are essential for the metabolism of macronutrients and to produce ATP. Micronutrients include vitamins and minerals, which are required in small amounts for proper bodily function.

Finally, hydration is critical for energy production as well. Dehydration can cause fatigue and decreased physical and mental performance, as water is necessary for many metabolic processes in the body. Water is also important for regulating body temperature and for maintaining proper blood flow to the muscles and organs.

To optimize energy production, it is important to consume a balanced diet that includes all three macronutrients and a variety of micronutrients. Additionally, staying properly hydrated by drinking water throughout the day can help to support energy levels and overall health.

Stress and sleep can both have a significant impact on energy levels.

Stress can be both physical and psychological, and both types of stress can lead to fatigue and decreased energy levels. Physical stress from over-exertion or injury can lead to muscle fatigue and decreased endurance, while psychological stress can lead to mental fatigue and decreased concentration. Stress also triggers the release of cortisol, a hormone that can increase blood sugar levels and lead to a burst of energy but can also cause fatigue and exhaustion over time.

Sleep is also critical for energy levels, as it is during sleep that the body repairs and restores itself. Lack of sleep or poor sleep quality can lead to daytime fatigue, decreased concentration, and decreased physical performance. This is because during sleep, the body produces ATP, the molecule that provides energy to cells, and repairs and restores tissues and organs that are essential for energy production.

Both stress and poor sleep quality can lead to an increase in the production of the hormone cortisol, which can interfere with the body's natural energy production processes. Additionally, stress and poor sleep quality can lead to unhealthy eating habits, such as overeating or consuming high-sugar foods, which can contribute to energy crashes and decreased performance.

To optimize energy levels, it is important to manage stress through techniques such as meditation, yoga, or deep breathing exercises, and to prioritize getting adequate, quality sleep each night. This can help support the body's natural energy production processes and promote overall health and well-being.

Maintaining optimal energy levels requires a multi-faceted approach, including proper nutrition, hydration, and physical activity. Here are some tips for optimizing energy levels:

Eat a balanced diet

Eating a well-balanced diet that includes complex carbohydrates, lean protein, healthy fats, and plenty of fruits and vegetables can help provide the body with the nutrients it needs to produce energy. Complex carbohydrates, such as whole grains and vegetables, provide sustained energy, while protein helps build and repair tissues. Healthy fats, such as those found in nuts, seeds, and avocado, also provide energy and support brain function.

Stay hydrated

Dehydration can lead to fatigue and decreased energy levels. Drinking plenty of water throughout the day can help ensure that the body is properly hydrated, which is essential for optimal energy production.

Get regular physical activity

Regular physical activity can help improve energy levels by promoting circulation, increasing endurance, and boosting mood. Even moderate physical activity, such as walking or cycling, can have a positive impact on energy levels.

Manage stress

Chronic stress can lead to fatigue and exhaustion, so it is important to find ways to manage stress levels. Techniques such as meditation, yoga, or deep breathing exercises can help reduce stress and promote relaxation.

Prioritize sleep

Getting adequate, quality sleep each night is essential for energy production and overall health. Aim for 7-8 hours of sleep per night and establish a regular sleep routine to help promote quality sleep.

Limit caffeine and sugar intake

While caffeine and sugar can provide a quick burst of energy, they can also lead to energy crashes and decreased performance. Limiting caffeine and sugar intake, especially later in the day, can help maintain steady energy levels throughout the day.

By incorporating these tips into your daily routine, you can help maintain optimal energy levels and promote overall health and well-being.

Digestion and its impact on health and fitness

The digestive process is the series of events that break down food into smaller components that the body can absorb and utilize for energy and other functions. The digestive system consists of various organs, including the mouth, esophagus, stomach, small intestine, large intestine, pancreas, liver, and gallbladder. Here is an overview of the digestive process and its role in nutrient absorption:

Mouth

The digestive process begins in the mouth, where food is chewed and mixed with saliva. Saliva contains enzymes that start to break down carbohydrates.

Esophagus

After being chewed, food is swallowed and passes through the esophagus, a muscular tube that connects the mouth to the stomach.

Stomach

In the stomach, food is mixed with digestive juices, including hydrochloric acid and enzymes that break down proteins. The stomach also grinds and churns the food into a thick liquid called chyme.

Small intestine

The small intestine is where most of the nutrients from food are absorbed into the bloodstream. The chyme from the stomach is mixed with digestive juices from the pancreas and liver, which help break down fats and carbohydrates. The small intestine also contains small finger-like projections called villi, which increase the surface area for nutrient absorption.

Large intestine

The large intestine absorbs water and electrolytes from the remaining food waste, forming solid feces.

Rectum and anus

The solid feces are stored in the rectum until they are eliminated from the body through the anus.

Nutrient absorption occurs primarily in the small intestine, where nutrients are absorbed into the bloodstream and transported to the body's cells for energy and other functions. Carbohydrates are broken down into simple sugars, which are absorbed into the bloodstream and transported to the liver. Fats are broken down into fatty acids and glycerol and transported to the liver for processing. Proteins are broken down into amino acids and also absorbed into the bloodstream.

The digestive process and nutrient absorption are critical for providing the body with the nutrients it needs to function properly. A healthy diet with a variety of nutrient-dense foods is essential for optimal digestive function and nutrient absorption.

Stress, hydration, and food choices can all have an impact on digestion.

Here's how each one can affect the digestive process:

Stress

When you're stressed, your body's "fight or flight" response is triggered, which can slow down digestion. Stress can also lead to changes in gut bacteria, which can affect digestive function. Additionally, stress can cause changes in eating habits, such as overeating or skipping meals, which can further disrupt digestion.

Hydration

Adequate hydration is important for maintaining healthy digestion. When you're dehydrated, your body can't produce enough saliva or digestive juices to break down food properly. This can lead to constipation, bloating, and other digestive issues. Drinking enough water and other fluids can help keep your digestive system functioning properly.

Food choices

The foods you eat can also have an impact on digestion. A diet high in processed and fried foods, sugar, and saturated fats can slow down digestion and lead to constipation and other digestive issues. On the other hand, a diet rich in fiber, fruits and vegetables, whole grains, and lean proteins can promote healthy digestion and regular bowel movements.

In addition to these factors, certain medical conditions and medications can also affect digestion. If you're experiencing persistent digestive issues, it's important to talk to your healthcare provider to determine the underlying cause and develop an appropriate treatment plan.

Here are some tips for improving digestion:

Eat slowly and mindfully

Eating too quickly and not chewing food thoroughly can lead to digestive issues. Taking the time to chew your food well and eat slowly can help your body digest food more easily.

Stay hydrated

Drinking enough water and fluids is important for maintaining healthy digestion. Aim for at least 8 glasses of water per day and try to drink fluids throughout the day.

Incorporate probiotics

Probiotics are beneficial bacteria that can help promote healthy digestion. They can be found in fermented foods like yogurt, kefir, sauerkraut, and kimchi, or taken as a supplement.

Eat fiber-rich foods

Fiber helps promote regular bowel movements and can improve digestive health. Good sources of fiber include fruits and vegetables, whole grains, legumes, and nuts.

Avoid trigger foods

Certain foods can trigger digestive issues, such as bloating, gas, and diarrhea. Common trigger foods include spicy foods, high-fat foods, and foods high in sugar. Keep track of what you eat and how it affects your digestion, and try to avoid trigger foods.

Exercise regularly

Regular exercise can help keep your digestive system healthy by promoting regular bowel movements and reducing stress.

Manage stress

Stress can have a negative impact on digestion. Practicing stress-reducing techniques like meditation, yoga, or deep breathing can help improve digestion.

If you're experiencing persistent digestive issues, it's important to talk to your healthcare provider to determine the underlying cause and develop an appropriate treatment plan.

Stress and its impact on health and fitness

Stress can have significant impacts on both physical and mental health. When we experience stress, our bodies release a hormone called cortisol, which triggers the body's fight-or-flight response. While this response can be helpful in short-term situations, chronic stress can lead to a range of negative health outcomes, including:

Increased risk of chronic diseases

Chronic stress has been linked to an increased risk of a range of chronic diseases, including heart disease, diabetes, and autoimmune disorders.

Weakened immune system

Stress can weaken the immune system, making it more difficult for the body to fight off infections and illnesses.

Digestive issues

Stress can impact digestion by causing symptoms like nausea, diarrhea, and constipation.

Sleep problems

Stress can also interfere with sleep, leading to issues like insomnia and sleep disturbances.

Mental health problems

Chronic stress is a risk factor for a range of mental health problems, including anxiety, depression, and burnout.

Physical symptoms

Stress can also lead to physical symptoms like headaches, muscle tension, and fatigue.

Managing stress is important for both physical and mental health. Some strategies for managing stress include:

- Practicing relaxation techniques like deep breathing, meditation, or yoga.
- Exercising regularly, which can help reduce stress levels and improve mood.
- Maintaining a healthy lifestyle with a balanced diet and adequate sleep.
- Seeking support from friends, family, or a mental health professional.
- Taking breaks and setting boundaries to prevent burnout.
- Identifying and avoiding stress triggers whenever possible.

There are different types of stress that people may experience, including acute and chronic stress.

Acute stress is a short-term response to a specific situation, such as a deadline at work or a sudden event like a car accident. This type of stress typically lasts for a brief period and can often be beneficial, helping us to respond quickly and effectively to the situation.

Chronic stress, on the other hand, is a type of stress that persists over a longer period, sometimes for months or years. It may result from ongoing issues like financial problems, work-related stress, or relationship difficulties. Chronic stress can be harmful to both physical and mental health and can lead to a range of negative health outcomes over time.

Chronic stress may cause the body to release higher levels of stress hormones like cortisol over a prolonged period, which can have negative effects on the body. This type of stress has been linked to an increased risk of chronic diseases like heart disease and diabetes, as well as mental health problems like depression and anxiety.

It's important to manage both acute and chronic stress to maintain good health. Strategies for managing acute stress may include deep breathing, taking a break, or seeking support from others. Managing chronic stress may involve making lifestyle changes like increasing physical activity or seeking professional support from a therapist or counselor.

Stress can affect many different aspects of our physical and mental health, including appetite, digestion, hormone levels, and sleep. Here are some of the ways that stress can impact these areas:

Stress can affect appetite in different ways. Some people may experience an increase in appetite and cravings for high-fat and high-sugar foods when they are stressed. Others may experience a decrease in appetite and may not feel like eating at all.

Stress can also affect digestion by causing changes in the way that the digestive system functions. For example, stress can cause the stomach to produce more acid, which can lead to heartburn and other digestive issues. It can also cause the muscles in the digestive tract to contract more, which can lead to diarrhea or constipation.

Stress can also impact hormone levels in the body. When we are stressed, the body releases hormones like cortisol and adrenaline to help us cope with the situation. Over time, chronic stress can lead to higher levels of cortisol in the body, which can disrupt the balance of other hormones like estrogen and testosterone.

Finally, stress can also impact sleep. When we are stressed, it can be harder to fall asleep and stay asleep throughout the night. This can lead to feelings of fatigue and exhaustion during the day, which can make it harder to cope with stress.

Overall, stress can have a significant impact on our physical and mental health. It's important to take steps to manage stress effectively, such as practicing relaxation techniques like deep breathing or meditation, engaging in regular physical activity, and seeking support from friends, family, or a mental health professional when needed.

Stress is a common experience for many individuals, and it can impact both physical and mental health.

While some level of stress can be helpful for motivation and productivity, chronic stress can have negative effects on the body and mind. Here are some tips for managing stress:

Mindfulness meditation is a technique that involves focusing on the present moment, without judgment. This practice can help to reduce stress by promoting relaxation and reducing negative thoughts.

Yoga is a physical practice that involves a series of postures and breathing exercises. It can help to reduce stress by promoting relaxation and reducing tension in the body.

Regular physical activity can help to reduce stress by promoting the release of endorphins, which are natural mood boosters. Additionally, physical activity can help to reduce tension and promote relaxation.

Deep breathing exercises can help to reduce stress by promoting relaxation and reducing tension in the body. One technique is to take deep breaths in through the nose and out through the mouth, focusing on the sensation of the breath.

Cognitive-behavioral therapy (CBT) is a type of talk therapy that focuses on changing negative thought patterns and behaviors. It can be helpful for managing stress and anxiety.

Poor time management can lead to stress and anxiety. To manage stress, it can be helpful to prioritize tasks and activities, and to set realistic goals and deadlines.

Having a support network can be helpful for managing stress. This may include friends, family members, or a therapist.

Practicing self-care can help to reduce stress and promote

relaxation. This may include activities such as taking a relaxing bath, practicing yoga, or reading a book.

By incorporating these tips into your routine, you can manage stress and promote overall health and well-being.

Strategies for Improving Sleep, Hunger, Recovery, Energy, Digestion, and Stress

Improving sleep, hunger, recovery, energy, digestion, and stress are essential for overall health and well-being. Here are some strategies that can help:

Sleep

- Establish a consistent sleep routine by going to bed and waking up at the same time each day.

- Create a sleep-conducive environment by keeping the room dark, quiet, and cool.
- Avoid caffeine and alcohol before bedtime.
- Limit screen time before bed, as the blue light emitted by electronic devices can disrupt sleep.
- Engage in relaxing activities before bed, such as reading or taking a warm bath.

Hunger

- Eat slowly and mindfully, paying attention to hunger and fullness cues.

- Focus on nutrient-dense foods, including fruits, vegetables, whole grains, lean proteins, and healthy fats.
- Stay hydrated by drinking plenty of water throughout the day.
- Incorporate fiber-rich foods, such as beans, nuts, seeds, and whole grains, into the diet to help promote feelings of fullness.

Recovery

- Incorporate rest days into your exercise routine to allow for proper recovery.
- Stay hydrated by drinking plenty of water throughout the day.
- Eat nutrient-dense foods that can help support recovery, such as lean proteins, complex carbohydrates, and healthy fats.
- Get adequate sleep to support physical and mental recovery.

Energy

- Eat a balanced diet that includes complex carbohydrates, lean proteins, and healthy fats to support energy levels.
- Stay hydrated by drinking plenty of water throughout the day.
- Engage in regular physical activity to help boost energy levels.
- Limit caffeine and sugar intake, as they can lead to energy crashes.

Digestion

- Eat slowly and mindfully, chewing food thoroughly before swallowing.
- Stay hydrated by drinking plenty of water throughout the day.
- Incorporate probiotics and fiber-rich foods, such as yogurt, kefir, sauerkraut, beans, nuts, seeds, and whole grains, into the diet to support healthy digestion.
- Avoid processed and high-fat foods, which can be difficult to digest.

Stress

- Engage in relaxation techniques, such as deep breathing, meditation, or yoga, to help manage stress.
- Exercise regularly, as physical activity can help reduce stress.
- Prioritize self-care activities, such as taking a bath, reading a book, or spending time with friends and family.
- Practice time-management techniques, such as making a to-do list or prioritizing tasks, to help reduce stress.

Overall, improving sleep, hunger, recovery, energy, digestion, and stress requires a holistic approach that involves incorporating healthy lifestyle habits into your daily routine. By prioritizing these areas of health, you can enhance your overall well-being and improve your quality of life.

Develop a Plan

Creating a personalized plan for improving health and fitness is crucial for achieving long-term success. No two individuals are the same, and everyone has unique needs and goals when it comes to their health and fitness journey. A personalized plan takes into consideration an individual's lifestyle, preferences, and health status, which ensures that the plan is both achievable and sustainable.

The first step in creating a personalized plan is to identify specific goals. These goals can be related to sleep, hunger, recovery, energy, digestion, and stress or any other aspect of health and fitness that the individual wants to improve. Setting specific, measurable, achievable, relevant, and time-bound (SMART) goals helps to establish a clear direction and provides motivation to work towards achieving them.

Once the goals are established, the next step is to identify the most effective strategies to achieve them. This involves identifying the underlying factors that are contributing to the individual's current status and developing strategies to address these factors. For example, if an individual has trouble sleeping, strategies such as establishing a regular sleep routine, creating a comfortable sleep environment, and limiting caffeine and screen time before bed can be effective.

It is also important to consider an individual's lifestyle and preferences when developing a plan. For example, if an individual dislikes running, then incorporating other forms of physical activity that they enjoy, such as swimming or cycling, can help to ensure consistency and enjoyment in their fitness routine. Similarly, if an individual has a busy work schedule, then identifying time-efficient workouts or meal prep strategies can help to ensure that their health and fitness goals fit within their schedule.

Creating a personalized plan is not a one-time event. It is important to regularly assess progress towards the goals, adjust strategies as needed, and establish new goals once the initial ones have been achieved. It is also important to recognize that setbacks can occur, and it is important to view them as learning opportunities rather than failures.

Overall, creating a personalized plan for improving health and fitness based on individual needs and goals is a critical step in achieving long-term success. By identifying specific goals, addressing underlying factors, and considering lifestyle and preferences, individuals can develop effective strategies that are achievable and sustainable, leading to improved health and well-being.

Conclusion

The interconnectedness of sleep, hunger, recovery, energy, digestion, and stress in health and fitness cannot be overstated. These factors all play a significant role in our overall physical and mental health and are intimately linked in complex ways.

Sleep is crucial for physical and mental health, as it allows the body to rest and repair. Sleep deprivation can lead to hormonal imbalances, increased appetite, and decreased energy levels, all of which can have negative impacts on health and fitness. The different stages of sleep all serve important functions in the body, including memory consolidation and cellular repair.

Hunger and appetite are regulated by hormones such as ghrelin and leptin. Proper nutrition, hydration, and stress management can all impact hunger cues and the body's ability to regulate appetite. Consuming nutrient-dense foods and staying hydrated can also support optimal energy production and recovery, further emphasizing the interconnectedness of these factors.

Recovery is essential for physical and mental health, and there are different types of recovery, including active and passive recovery. Stress, sleep, and nutrition can all impact recovery, highlighting the importance of taking a holistic approach to health and fitness.

Energy is necessary for physical activity and overall health, and it is influenced by macronutrients, micronutrients, and hydration. Stress and sleep can also impact energy levels, underscoring the importance of managing stress and maintaining good sleep hygiene.

Digestion plays a critical role in nutrient absorption, and stress, hydration, and food choices can all impact digestion. By eating slowly and mindfully, staying hydrated, and incorporating probiotics and fiber-rich foods into the diet, individuals can improve their digestive health and overall well-being.

Finally, stress can have significant impacts on physical and mental health, including digestion, energy levels, and sleep quality. Managing stress through techniques such as mindfulness meditation, yoga, and regular physical activity can be beneficial in supporting overall health and fitness.

The interconnectedness of sleep, hunger, recovery, energy, digestion, and stress highlights the importance of taking a holistic approach to health and fitness. By prioritizing these factors and developing a personalized plan, individuals can achieve optimal health and well-being.